BODYBUILDING AND STEROIDS: MY PERSONAL STORY

BY

PAUL NAM

For more works by this author, please visit:

www.theworkoutloft.com/linkshop

OTHER BOOKS BY THE AUTHOR

FAT TO FIT IN 8 WEEKS

SCRAWNY TO BRAWNY IN 8 WEEKS

NUTRITION 101: BUILDING THE FOUNDATION

IMMUNE SYSTEM 8: BOOST YOUR IMMUNE SYSTEM NATURALLY

IT'S ALL ABOUT YOUR HEALTH: FOOD RECIPES

THE BOOK OF CHOICES: THE LIVES OF 2 ATHLETES

THE ULTIMATE GUIDE TO CORE(ABS) TRAINING: NO MORE LOW BACK PAIN

DUMBBELL TRAINING: FOR MEN AND WOMEN

LEARN HOW TO STRETCH: FOR BETTER MOVEMENT AND HEALTH

DUMBBELL AND CORE(ABS) TRAINING COMBINED

BEGINNER'S GUIDE TO DIET AND TRAINING

TABLE OF CONTENTS

INTRODUCTION

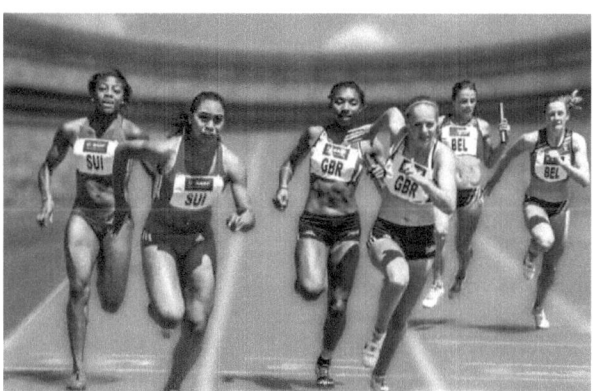

The competition date has arrived. You have slept, ate, and trained all year for this race. First place is a Nike endorsement, television exposure, and $100,000. You approach the start line while taking a deep breath and quickly glance over at the other seven contestants. Ready, start, go! The gun goes off, and you explode upwards as you run towards the finish line. You feel the rush of adrenaline surge through your body as the finish line is in sight. One guy keeps gaining on you no matter how hard you run. You finished second place and gave everything you had, but that one guy was just faster. Your coach and trainer had suggested a Winstrol cycle to enhance recovery and speed at the beginning of the season, but you wanted to do this competition without any drugs. Now that suggestion didn't seem such a bad idea.

This situation is why athletes use steroids and other performance-enhancing drugs to win. With any competition comes the prestige of winning first place and everything that comes with it. Bodybuilders use steroids and other drugs to look big, ripped, and powerful. Olympic and other athletes use performance- enhancing drugs to have better endurance, be faster, and to be stronger.

Even if the top level athletes and bodybuilders decided not to use performance-enhancing drugs, they would still be faster or bigger than the average person. It is their genetics that makes them champions from the start. Mike Phelps is an example of a genetic freak. His hands look like webs, and he is double jointed in many parts of his arms and legs, so that gives him an advantage as a swimmer.

Welcome to Bodybuilding and Anabolic Steroids: My Personal Story. This is my story of what it took to become a national level bodybuilder and to put on 55 lbs of muscle on a 5'8' frame.

BODYBUILDING HISTORY

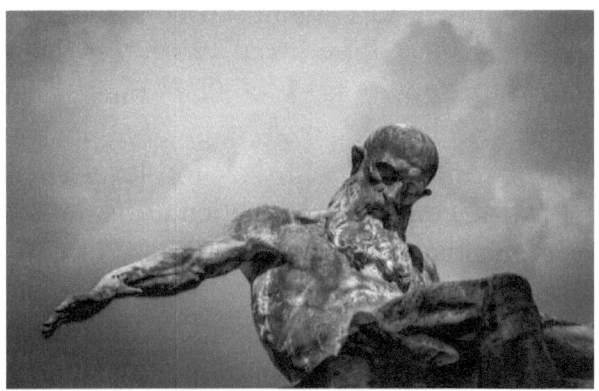

The front double bicep pose, rear lat spread pose, and the side chest pose. These are the three poses that make up the seven compulsory poses in a bodybuilding competition. Some people often wonder what bodybuilding is? Bodybuilding is defined as the use of resistance exercise to control and develop one's muscularity. Eugene Sandow was the first person to promote bodybuilding shortly after the 19th century. He then organized the first ever bodybuilding competition in September 1901, and it was a huge success. Today, there are many thousands of competitions all over the world, and the most prestigious and recognized competition held for bodybuilding is the Mr. Olympia.

The first Mr. Olympia competition was held on September 18, 1965, in New York. This competition was created by Joe Weider, and this enabled the Mr. Universe winners to continue to compete and earn money doing what they loved. With the first-place prize money now at $400,000 plus company endorsements, there is no shortage of athletes trying to claim this title. As with any top-level sport, the winners all have superior genetics to begin with, so the average person cannot reach this level no matter what drugs they use.

Millions of people around the world today are involved in the art of bodybuilding and the fitness lifestyle. Most people are into this type of lifestyle to be healthy, both mentally and physically. Working out, whether it be resistance training or cardiovascular training, is healthy for the mind and body. The pioneers of this sport were John Grimek, Eugene Sandow, Steeve Reeves, Bill Pearl, and Reg Park. Even with limited knowledge and basic training equipment, they sculpted their physiques to an impressive level. Bodybuilding training equipment has evolved since the 1900's, but nothing will ever surpass the basic dumbbell and barbell for hardcore training.

Bodybuilding competitions today are a multi-million-dollar business. Various organizations such as the World Natural Bodybuilding Federation (WNBF) and the International Federation of Bodybuilding and Fitness (IFBB) run bodybuilding and fitness shows across the world. If bodybuilding never existed, organizations like these would never have been developed. Smaller organizations like the Ontario Physique Association (OPA) allow the general public to compete in bodybuilding and fitness shows. Some people find out they have the genetics, money, mentality, and self-discipline to achieve professional status and compete around the world. As with any high-level competition, it is the edge to win at all costs. However, to become bigger, better, and to look like a freak requires drugs.

PERFORMANCE ENHANCING DRUGS

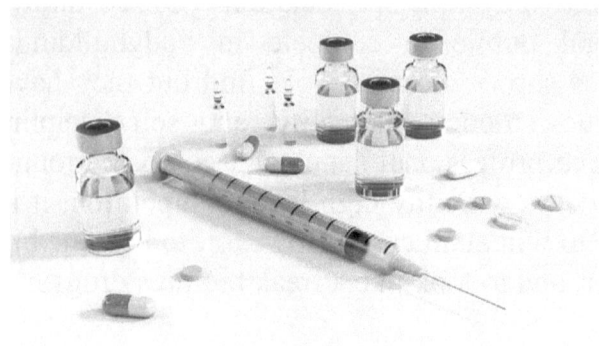

Steroids, growth hormone and clenbuterol are examples of performance- enhancing drugs that are used by athletes and bodybuilders. These drugs can be used for either performance or to obtain a certain look as we see in today's bodybuilding. Most bodybuilders have a certain walk that defines them. They can be seen walking with their elbows out, head up, and lats wide out. In the Olympics, drugs are evident and can be seen through the inhuman performance. In bodybuilding competitions, drugs are evident through the inhuman muscle mass the contestants possess. If a large female bodybuilder shaved her head, it would be a challenge to know if she was a female or not. Not every bodybuilder and athlete uses drugs, but for the most part, it is no secret to the public. Athletes like Lance Armstrong and Jose Conseco have admitted to taking performance- enhancing drugs. Let's not forget about Ben Johnson who was caught using Winstrol and was stripped of his medal in 1988 at the Los Angeles Olympic Games. When a person takes drugs such as steroids, they get increased strength, mass, recovery, and speed. As good as that sounds, what they also get is unwanted side effects. For this chapter, I will be going over the most popular types of performance- enhancing drugs and the side effects that are associated with them.

Let's start with the most popular and widely used drug in bodybuilding and in sports, anabolic steroids. In the year of 1931, a German chemist named Adolf Butenandt was the first person to purify the hormone, androstenone. He managed to extract this hormone from a few litres of urine, and this was the beginning and birth of anabolic steroids. Who thought urine would be the start of a synthetic hormone that would soon change the entire world? Throughout this chapter, I will discuss steroids such as Testosterone, Winstrol, Trenbolone, Dianabol, Anavar, and Decca Durabolin.

First on the list is testosterone. Testosterone is a very important hormone for both men and women and is needed for the proper functioning of the human body. It is a very powerful hormonc and is classified as either androgenic or anabolic. Androgenic is any steroid hormone that promotes male development and characteristics, while anabolic is defined as the process of building up the materials of living tissue. Testosterone is responsible for the development of the testicles, prostate, muscle tissue, bone density, and strength. Most men use testosterone for hormone replacement therapy or to increase levels above normal for performance enhancement purposes. Testosterone also enhances recovery time and red blood cell count giving the user greater endurance. This hormone is available for use in four different forms: a water base, pill, gel, and oil base form. The oil base injectable forms are called testosterone propionate, ethanate, cypionate, Sustanon 250, and omnadren. The water base injectable form is called testosterone suspension. The gel and pill form are used in testosterone replacement therapy (TRT) along with injectable testosterone ethanate and cypionate. Abuse of this hormone can cause the user some adverse effects. Some side effects are water retention, acne, hair loss, natural testosterone suppression, high blood pressure, testicular shrinkage, and a change in HDL/LDL levels. The long-acting testosterone esters such as ethanate and cypionate are often used in a bulking cycle as they cause water retention. The short- acting testosterone esters such as propionate and suspension are used during a cutting cycle as they tend to cause less water retention. Sustanon 250 and omnadren are unique as they both have long and short- acting testosterone esters inside of them. I have used every type of testosterone whether it is for a bulking or a cutting cycle. I have felt all the side effects associated with them, but I kept my dosages fairly safe as I never went over 1000 mg. My top dosage was 900 mg, and that pushed my body weight up to 205lbs. I had no neck, was eating over 5000 calories a day, and was lifting tremendous amounts of weights. Was I healthy? No, I was not, but extreme bodybuilding has nothing to do with health. It is all about being as big as possible, and I will talk about this more in the upcoming chapters. I will not be going over injection protocols and timing for any of these drugs as my intentions are not to teach people how to use them.

Winstrol is the next drug to discuss, and everyone knows the story about Ben Johnson. He was caught using Winstrol in the 1988 Olympics and was stripped of his medal. Winstrol was first developed by Winthrop Laboratories in the late 1950's and is also known as Stanozolol. This steroid is considered anabolic and is one of the preferred drugs to use when a person is preparing for a bodybuilding or fitness competition. Winstrol is also a favourite for competitive athletes because of its abilities to promote strength and endurance without the unwanted bulk. As with most steroids, Winstrol will enhance protein synthesis and increase nitrogen retention inside of the muscles. This is why bodybuilders can ingest 300-500 grams of protein a day when they are on a steroid cycle. Winstrol comes in an injectable water base form and a pill form. This steroid is fast acting meaning the effects are seen faster than long- acting ester steroids like Decca Durabolin. Winstrol has many side effects and is toxic to the liver. The side effects of this drug are testosterone suppression, joint pain, acne, hair loss, and increased blood pressure. I have used both forms of Winstrol many times during my contest preparation and noticed a strong decrease in my libido. This was not a great feeling at all. This steroid worked well for my cutting cycles as I would often combine it with other cutting agents. My longest cycle on Winstrol was 6 weeks, and I did notice some joint pain (elbows), but that stopped after I discontinued the steroid.

Trenbolone is one of the most powerful and versatile anabolic steroids on the market today. This steroid was created in 1960 and was first introduced as Finajet. In 1980, finaplex pellets were created in order to increase the tissue in cattle before they were slaughtered. These pellets are now used by athletes and bodybuilders to enhance performance or muscle mass. Trenbolone is classified as both androgenic and anabolic. This makes it a very versatile steroid that can be used in both a bulking or cutting cycle. Trenbolone is one of the most popular and widely used steroids on the market today. The two forms of trenbolone are called acetate and ethanate. Ethanate is the long-acting form, and the acetate is the short-acting form. This means ethanate would require fewer injections weekly as it has a greater half-life versus the acetate. The acetate would have to be injected more frequently since it has a shorter life span. Side effects from trenbolone may include gynecomastia, acne, hair loss, increased LDL, decreased HDL, testosterone suppression, and increased aggression. I have used all forms of trenbolone (finaplex, finajet) in order to get ready for my bodybuilding shows and during the offseason. After a few injections, I could see and notice a difference in my strength and muscle hardness. I also noticed my aggression was becoming uncontrollable and I will go over this in more detail in the upcoming chapters.

Dianabol is definitely one of the most popular oral steroids in today's market. While some steroids were created for the use of medical benefits, Dianabol was created solely for enhancement purposes. Dr. Ziegler was the first person to create this steroid after he learned how the Soviets were using testosterone in the Olympics. Dianabol is also known as methandrostenolone and is considered androgenic, but it's known to have some anabolic properties as well. This steroid is used primarily in a mass and strength cycle. Dianabol comes in both oral and injectable form, but the oral form is the most popular. This steroid is known to enhance three things: protein synthesis, nitrogen retention, and glycogenolysis. As good as this may be, the side effects are not pleasant. The side effects may include increased LDL cholesterol (bad), increased blood pressure, water retention, testosterone suppression, and liver toxicity. Dianabol is a fast-acting steroid, so pills or injections are taken more frequently. I have used this steroid during my off-season cycles, and the end result was a good amount of muscle mass. One thing I really noticed was how puffy my muscles looked when combining Dianabol with testosterone since both cause water retention.

Another popular oral steroid to dominate the industry is Anavar. This steroid is used by both men and women because it carries fewer side effects than most steroids. Anavar is anabolic in nature and also is known as Oxandrolone. This steroid was created in 1960 by a company called G.D. Searle and is used for many types of medical treatment plans. Doctors prescribe this steroid for the purpose of weight gain after surgery or after severe weight loss. Anavar is also used for the treatment of osteoporosis, hepatitis, and for promoting growth in children who have hormone dysfunction. Bodybuilders and athletes use this drug during a cutting cycle or for athletic enhancement. Anavar will create lean muscle growth, fat loss, increased strength, and increased muscular endurance. The side effects associated with this drug are usually mild but can include acne, hair loss, change in HDL/LDL cholesterol levels, testosterone suppression, and liver toxicity. Anavar is a fast- acting steroid that comes in a pill or capsule form and must be taken daily. I did not use much Anavar during my competition days but used it more when I was training in MMA to enhance my athletic performance. I noticed how good my cardiovascular workouts were and did not notice many side effects other than mild testosterone suppression.

The last steroid on the list to review is Decca Durabolin. Decca Durabolin first appeared on the market in 1962 by a company called Organon. This steroid is considered anabolic and is commonly used by athletes for its performance enhancement attributes. Bodybuilders use Decca during a bulking cycle, and one unique quality this steroid has is the ability to provide joint relief by enhancing collagen synthesis. This steroid is used in the medical industry for the treatment of osteoporosis, muscle wasting diseases, anemia, and certain forms of breast cancer. Decca comes in a liquid form so it must be injected and is a slow-acting steroid. This steroid will enhance nitrogen balance, increase muscle mass slowly, enhance muscular endurance, and enhance overall recovery. The side effects from Decca are gynecomastia, high blood pressure, acne, hair loss, negative change in HDL/LDL cholesterol levels, and testosterone suppression. Decca was one of my favourite steroids to use while on a heavy testosterone cycle because of its ability to provide an extra joint cushion for my heavy training. I did notice some testosterone suppression, and when I combined it with Dianabol, my blood pressure would increase. This usually resulted in several nose bleeds a day.

We will now go over another very popular performance enhancing drug called Human Growth Hormone. HGH is a protein hormone produced by our pituitary gland. The use of HGH was first seen in 1958 and after a year, the US FDA banned its use for the general public. Human growth hormone is one of the most important hormones in the human body as it can affect our skeletal muscle, bones, and internal organs. Real HGH comes in an injectable form and can be very expensive. This hormone must frequently be injected since the half-life is very short. Growth hormone can take up to 8-12 weeks before any positive results can be seen in terms of fat loss. Athletes and bodybuilders use HGH together with anabolic steroids, and using it alone will not promote massive growth or performance. If used by itself, HGH will enhance recovery and have a positive effect on the metabolism. In the medical field, doctors use growth hormone to treat dwarfism, people with HIV and HGH deficiency, burn victims, and muscle wasting conditions. This hormone is hailed as an anti-aging drug and can be used in the United States under doctor supervision as growth hormone therapy. Did you ever notice how muscular the men on the American police force are compared to the Canadian police force? Though this hormone is relatively safe and is not a foreign substance in the body, abusing HGH will cause side effects. More common side effects are water retention, joint pain, and headaches. More adverse side effects are enlarged hands, feet, jaw, and growth of the internal organs. The next time you watch a Mr. Olympia, look at their stomachs when they stand relaxed. Their stomachs actually stick out from all the internal organ growth. I have used HGH for my bulking and cutting cycles, and one thing I did notice was the mind blowing pumps from combining HGH, steroids, and eating over 5000 calories. One serious side effect I noticed, however, was the growth in my jaw and elbows. It became so bad I became paranoid to take pictures of my face. After stopping HGH, all the abnormal growth went away after a few months.

Bodybuilders and athletes do use other performance-enhancing drugs other than anabolic steroids. I call these categories auxiliary drugs as they are needed to balance out what is put inside of the body or to amplify the results. Every year new drugs are produced, but I will go over the most popular ones such as Nolvadex, Clomid, Clenbuterol, Peptides, and human chorionic gonadotropin (HCG).

Nolvadex is one of the most commonly used anti-estrogens when a person is on anabolic steroids. This unique drug was created in 1961 and is also known as Tamoxifen Citrate. Nolvadex was first used to treat females with breast cancer, but then bodybuilders found another use for it as well. This drug works as an anti-estrogen by binding to the estrogen receptors in the place of estrogen. By attaching itself to the estrogen receptors, this prevents the estrogen hormone from performing its actions in various parts of the body. Nolvadex also has strong testosterone stimulating characteristics and works by blocking the negative feedback that is brought on by estrogen at the pituitary. This stimulates the release of extra Luteinizing Hormone (LH) and Follicle Stimulating Hormone (FSH). These two hormones are needed for testosterone production. Very little side effects have been reported, and this is a well-tolerated drug for both men and females. I have used Nolvadex at the end of most of my steroid cycles to help block excessive estrogen conversion and help to kick start my testosterone production. The longest I have used this drug is for 3-4 weeks, and I felt no side effects.

Clomid is another popular drug that is used in Post Cycle Therapy (PTC). Post cycle therapy is used at the end of a steroid cycle when a person is ready to come off their steroids. This drug was first recognized in the early 1970s and is also known as Clomiphene Citrate. Clomid is similar to Nolvadex as it is used to combat estrogenic side effects that are caused by anabolic steroids. It is also used in post cycle therapy to stimulate testosterone production after a steroid cycle has been discontinued. For bodybuilding usage, Clomid has the ability to stimulate the pituitary to release more LH and FSH, as this will stimulate natural testosterone production. Clomid has anti-estrogenic properties that are useful to bodybuilders who use anabolic steroids. When this drug is used, it has the ability to reduce water retention, gynecomastia, and high blood pressure. For medical purposes, Clomid is used as a fertility aid in females because of its ability to release gonadotropins. By releasing more gonadotropins in females, there is a greater chance of an egg being released. Side effects from this drug are rare but may cause abdominal cramping and hot flashes. I have used Clomid for all my post cycle therapy and have had some good results in getting a boost to my own natural testosterone production. The longest I used this drug was for a few weeks, and I felt no negative side effects.

One of the most commonly used drugs for fat burning is clenbuterol. This unique drug is a bronchodilator and is used to treat breathing disorders like asthma. Clenbuterol is mostly used by bodybuilders and physique athletes during their contest preparation. It is also a favourite for people who are looking to lose some body fat. Clenbuterol works by stimulating the sympathomimetic nervous system in the human body. By stimulating the beta-2 receptor, this reverses the air way obstructions and provides improved breathing for the users. This drug works by increasing the body's temperature, which enhances the metabolism and this causes the person to burn greater body fat. The side effects associated with this drug include jittery, shaky hands, muscle cramps, and increased sweating. The last side effect is quite obvious as when a person burns fat, they sweat. Some users have reported headaches, and excessive amounts can cause insomnia, high blood pressure, and irregular heartbeats. I have used clenbuterol to get ready for my bodybuilding shows and during the summer months to stay lean. I noticed some impressive fat loss when combining it with cardio and a clean diet. As for side effects, my dosages were kept reasonable, so I only experienced the jittery feeling. One time my legs did cramp so bad, I could not walk after a heavy cardio session. As a result, I almost fell over on the floor. How is that for looking cool at the gym?

As bodybuilders and athletes become bigger and faster, new drugs are constantly being used in pursuit of winning. One class of drugs that has caught the attention of athletes and bodybuilder are peptides. The peptides that are mentioned here are the ones that cause an increase in a person's growth hormone levels. They are GHRP-2, GHRP-6, Ipamorelin, and Hexarelin. Peptides are used by bodybuilders and athletes for their ability to aid in recovery, anti-aging, and fat loss. People often wonder what they are made of? Peptides are short-chain amino acids linked together by a peptide bond. Our bodies use these short chain amino acids to cause a surge in our existing growth hormone (GH).

Using real synthetic growth hormone can be costly, and people often use these peptides as a cheaper alternative. A cycle of synthetic growth hormone would cost over a thousand dollars versus spending a few hundred dollars on peptides. There are so many different types of peptides out there, so I am going to keep it as general as possible and mention them briefly. As with any drug, there are side effects. Some side effects are joint pain, headaches, bloating, and water retention. If you are going to use peptides, research them and know how to use them properly. I have used a few peptides for my bodybuilding shows and did notice how strong my immune system was while on them.

Last on the list is human chorionic gonadotropin which is known as HCG. This hormone was first seen in the market in 1920 and was sold as an extract. HCG is a polypeptide hormone that is found in pregnant women. This drug is used to treat various conditions like female infertility, low testosterone, and weight loss. HCG is commonly used during a steroid cycle or after the cycle has been discontinued. From the use of anabolic steroids, a person's natural testosterone production is suppressed. Once the steroid cycle has stopped, the natural testosterone production will start again. This process is very slow, and the user can lose muscle mass. In order to combat this condition, the user often implements a post cycle therapy (PTC) plan in order to speed up the recovery process. Most people use SERMS such as Nolvadex, Clomid, or Arimidex as part of their PTC plan. Some people often used HCG prior to using SERMS to further enhance the recovery process. Another good thing that comes from HCG use is the ability to keep the user's testicles full during a steroid cycle. The use of testosterone causes the person's testicles to shrink because their own testosterone production is being suppressed. The body is getting testosterone from another source, so it slows down its own natural supply. Thank goodness for HCG because no guy likes to have their testicles look like two raisins. The side effects from HCG are very rare but can cause such issue as headaches, rashes, or gastrointestinal issues. I have used HCG many times and have noticed testicular fullness while on it. Using it before Nolvadex did seem to increase the effectiveness of the SERM and did help speed up the recovery process.

THE MINDSET OF A BODYBUILDER

When we start to grow up, we often try to find an identity that will suit us. People who graduate from university become business owners, teachers, doctors, and some become competitive athletes or bodybuilders. People often wonder why a person would want to eat ten chicken breasts a day, inject themselves with steroids, and train until they throw up. The lifestyle of a hard-core bodybuilder is nothing but glamorous, and yet millions of people are addicted to the lifestyle. Some athletes choose to be natural while most choose to use performance-enhancing drugs. Some people just enjoy the bodybuilding lifestyle and choose not to compete. To compete takes ultimate discipline when it comes to the training and eating. Throughout this chapter, I hope to explain to you what goes on in the mind of a hard-core bodybuilder.

People who are seen at the gym are often categorized into two groups. One group is classified as the people who love training, and the other group only go because they know it is good for them. Any serious athlete or bodybuilder loves to be at the gym and is known as a gym rat. When a person first starts to resistance train, they usually see good changes in their body. They lose fat, build muscle, and start to feel good about themselves. For a male, they start to put on more muscle mass, and their clothes fit tighter. For a female, they start to lose body fat, and their clothes fit looser. These changes are very addictive and are what fuels the person to keep going. Most people are happy with small changes in their bodies and do not want to go any further. A few of those people choose to compete to see how much further they can go. When a person enters a show, they commit 10-12 weeks of their lives to eating, training, and using performance enhancing drugs. The 10-12 weeks is a physical and mental challenge but if the person does well in the competition, the reward is first place or top 3. If the person is placed within top 3 or wins, they are eligible to compete at a higher level. For most people, the dieting becomes easier as they know what to expect. Every time a person competes, their body gets used to the eating and training, and it becomes a normal pattern of behaviour. After my first show, I found it easier to eat clean, and soon it became a way of life.

The drugs also become addictive as the person gets used to the feeling of being pumped up all the time. The new look is also addictive as people often stare at the newly transformed human being at the gym and in everyday life. For those people who enjoy it, the whole process can change their life. Once a person has achieved that perfect physique, they often have a hard time letting that go. If you are a girl reading this, imagine every guy staring at you uncontrollably and commenting on how beautiful you look everywhere. If you are a guy reading this, imagine every girl coming up to you and telling you how gorgeous you are. As human beings, we thrive on attention from others. That is why feedback is so addictive as people like to see how many likes they get on their social media posts.

MY FIRST BODYBUILDING COMPETITION

Most stories start by describing how skinny and scrawny the writer was at age 14 so he started weightlifting to put on some muscle. Even though that is true in my case, let's jump right to when I competed in my first bodybuilding show at the age of 19. After learning how to eat properly, I successfully bulked up to a weight of 180 lbs, and at 5'8' I was no monster, but I had enough muscle to do my first show. My plan was to compete as a middleweight or lightweight, but since this was my first show, I had no idea how my body would respond to the diet, drugs, and training. If a person can drop 10 lbs of fat and maintain most of their muscle, they are doing well. I had to plan my competition cycle, and it would consist of Decca Durabolin, Sustanon 250, Testosterone Propionate, Finaplex, Clenbuterol, Nolvadex, and some diuretics. The whole process would be 10 weeks in length so the cycle would be 10 weeks. For the first 5 weeks, I would use Decca Durabolin and Sustanon 250 then I would switch to test propionate and finaplex for my last 5 weeks. I would run clenbuterol throughout the 9 weeks, and the last week I would use some diuretics and Nolvadex. The test propionate was stopped one week out, and the finaplex was used right up to the show. I am not going to get into dosages and frequency of what I took as this book is not about educating people on how to use steroids but just to tell my story.

Next came the fun part, the diet. I would have to follow a low carbohydrate, high protein, and low-fat diet. The diet is the most challenging part for most people if they love carbohydrates, fats, and salty foods. Basically, I would have to eat as clean as possible meaning no sugar, fats, and salt for 10 weeks. A cheat meal would be implemented once a week, so I would have something to look forward to.

The first few weeks were not too challenging as my body was getting used to the low carbohydrate diet. During the evening, I started to crave certain foods I would never usually eat. Foods like chocolate, chips, ice cream, and hot dogs. Watching the food commercials on television became agonizing torture as I wanted to eat all the tasty food on the TV screen. Every week, I would count down the days to my cheat meal which usually was on a Saturday. When Saturday came, I would stuff my face with pizza, ice cream, and chips. Afterwards, my stomach would hurt so I would lie down and rub my belly to relieve some of the indigestion. It didn't really work.

The Decca Durabolin and Sustanon kept my muscles full while I kept on the calorie restricted diet. I noticed some fat loss with the clenburatol, but my energy levels started to drop after a few weeks into the diet. When a person trains for a show, they must include cardiovascular workouts in order to lose body fat. I did not enjoy cardiovascular activities, and my one bodybuilder friend always told me to do more cardio. I cursed every time I saw the treadmill, bike, or elliptical. Throughout the 10 weeks, I had a national level bodybuilder help me through the process since this was my first show. Finding someone to help or coach you through the process is a good idea. This is crucial as most people think they can compete and just do it themselves. I started to learn all the mandatory poses and loved the posing. What guy doesn't like to pose and flex his muscles in front of a mirror or in front of some girls? Putting the ego aside, the posing was fun because I could see the changes in my muscles.

Once I switched over to the testosterone propionate and finaplex, my temper became an issue. I was literally starving my body, training like a maniac, and doing a large steroid cycle. My family, coworkers, and friends noticed how grumpy and bitchy I was becoming. When the clenbuterol and finaplex mixed together, it really started to affect my sleeping. I quickly learned how to use melatonin, valerian root, kava kava, and red wine. Combining red wine and melatonin seemed to knock me out cold for a good 5-6 hours. When I did sleep, the dreams were very violent as they would often include people chasing me with chainsaws and axes. I attribute these amazing dreams to finaplex as this is a powerful steroid that can make people crazy when abused.

As I entered my last two weeks, I could no longer enjoy my cheat meals, and this was not an easy thing to do. My weight was down to 169lbs, so I was on track. My energy levels were very low, and my sex drive was non-existent, so I lost interest in women. This was an odd feeling to me as I usually have a healthy appetite for the opposite sex. When my body fat level went below 8 percent, the last thing on my mind was having sex. At the gym, people were complimenting me on how great I looked but the last few weeks are the toughest for any bodybuilder as I just wanted to eat a cheeseburger and some ice cream.

For a bodybuilding competition, a competitor must put together a 60-90 second posing routine with some music of their choice. They must pick a song or mix that is suited to them and their posing routine. One of my best friends is a DJ, so I had no issue with the music. The first time I received my posing trunks, they looked like something a male stripper would wear. I had to be comfortable with wearing them so I tried them on for a few of my lady friends and they seemed to enjoy them for some reason. So I figured this is what bodybuilding competitions are all about, wearing a g string, flexing my muscles, and doing steroids.

The final week is the most crucial part as you need to figure out how to manipulate carbohydrates, fats, proteins, salt, potassium, and water. At this point, I cut out my testosterone propionate and clenbuterol but kept the finaplex to keep my muscles looking full. I would add in Nolvadex or Arimidex the last two weeks to give my muscles a harder look. What I used for my first show was minimal compared to what guys take today. My approach to steroids was to use as minimal as possible and then make the best gains possible with hard training and good nutrition. However, my mindset changed as I grew bigger and advanced in the bodybuilding shows.

I found the water manipulation very interesting as drinking two gallons of water for a few days was no easy feat. Sunday to Wednesday I would drink two gallons of water, and soon the washroom became my best friend. Thursday, I would cut it down to one gallon and then Friday, half a gallon. Saturday was the show date so there would be no water intake, just sips throughout the day. I took Aldactone, which is a potassium sparring diuretic, a few days out to help push out all the extra water inside of my body. The diuretics started to work as I noticed my skin was becoming thin and my cheek bones were starting to sink in from the fluid loss. The one thing I really noticed was the loss of brain power. From all the fluid loss, my brain wasn't working at full capacity. I weighed myself on Friday morning and noticed my weight changed from 164 lbs to 154 lbs from the Thursday night. A bodyweight drop of 10 lbs. On Friday night, my calves started to cramp uncontrollably so I stretched them out and took an anti-cramp supplement and it slowly went away.

The night before the show, I could not sleep due to being both nervous and excited. I was anxious to get this show over with, so I could be normal again. One interesting thing a competitor can do if they are depleted and lean enough the night before is to eat sugar, sodium, and fat. An example would be a piece of cheesecake and a slice of pizza. The theory behind this is to load the body full of fat and glycogen the night before, so when a person pumps with weights, the sugar and fat will go directly into the muscles. The muscles become super pumped and balloon up when they are on stage creating a fuller look. The process is called sugar and fat loading. I did not try this as I felt I was not lean enough, so I just ate a meal consisting of yams and chicken.

My first show was in Mississauga and was held at Meadowville Secondary School. Most bodybuilding and fitness shows are held in a school or auditorium as a stage is needed to showcase a person's physique. In a bodybuilding show, people are divided by weight classes. For the men, the weight classes are bantamweight, lightweight, middleweight, light heavy, heavyweight, and super heavyweight. My two close friends came up with me for support since it was my first show. I was entered into two different classes, junior bodybuilder, and men's lightweight bodybuilding. I could compete in the junior class since my age was only 19 so I had to take my chances in two different classes. The night before the show, the judges weigh all the competitors to see if they make their weight classes. My weight was 154lbs, so I was in the lightweight class. With a height of 5'8', I was not the biggest guy there, but my legs looked ripped, and my overall symmetry was balanced. I had no idea I would lose over 16 lbs and then drop another 10 lbs of water.

I looked around the room and noticed there were two other junior bodybuilders and eight other lightweight men. I knew this was going to be a battle and a long day. Other than being thirsty, tired, and hungry, I was happy to be here. The show is broken down into a morning and evening show. The morning show would be the compulsory poses and then the evening show would consist of the posing routine and the awards. As I ate some chocolate bars, my one friend helped me with my final touches of the spray tan. Bodybuilders and physique athletes must look at least two shades darker under the bright lights. If a person is not dark enough, the person will look white under the lights. Last came the posing oil and then the pump up. The posing oil is applied to highlight the muscle underneath the lights. The pump up process is pretty quick as I did some push ups, dumbbell back rows, and dumbbell side laterals. The sugar from the chocolate bars started to pump up my muscles, and I was ready for battle.

After posing, posing, and more posing, I was placed first in the junior class and third in the lightweight men's class. All the bad dreams, muscle cramps, and chicken breasts were worth it as I came home with two trophies. The first thing I wanted to do was to drink water, eat some good food, and then have a shower. No more chicken breasts, fish, steamed vegetables, or yams for a while. At the age of 19, I felt somewhat content as most of my friends were at clubs drinking and partying all night. This competition would set my career as a bodybuilder and a personal trainer. I would now have to figure out my game plan for level 2. Level 2 would require me to train harder, eat more food, and do more steroids.

QUICK TEST

Do you have what it takes to compete in a bodybuilding show? To determine if you have what it takes to compete in a bodybuilding or fitness show, answer the following questions with one of the following answers: yes, or no.

1. Are you able to eat a bland diet for 10-12 weeks and not lose your mind?

2. Do you have two thousand dollars to spend on the competition?

3. Do you have the ability to you push yourself through intense training even when you have no energy?

4. Can you drink two to three gallons of water a day for a week?

5. Can you function on an irregular sleep schedule?

If you answered no to any of the questions, pick another sport to compete in. Bodybuilding and fitness shows require a certain mindset in order to complete the whole process.

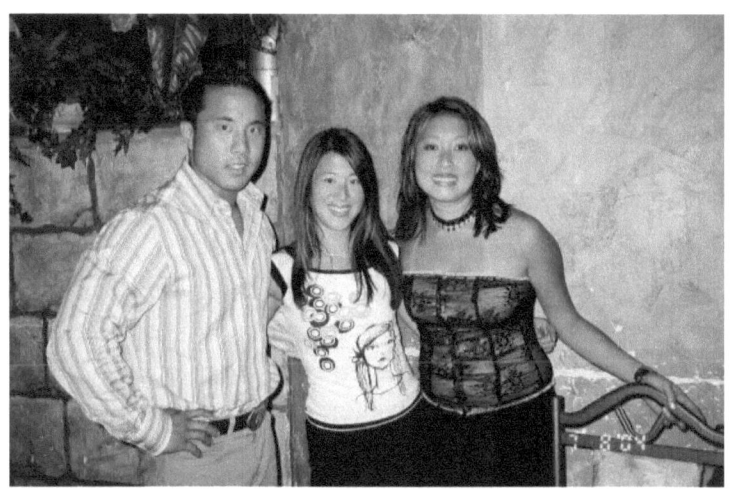

Bulked up to 190 lbs with my 2 sisters.

HOW I STARTED BODYBUILDING

My life started out in a small city called St. Catherine's which is located in the Niagara region. I arrived on this earth on September 24, 1978, making me 38 as I am writing this. I was the typical skinny, smart Asian kid growing up in a white suburban city. My family consisted of a mother, father, myself, and two older sisters. My one sister was a year older than me, so we fought quite a bit as most kids do. Since there was only a year age difference between us, we also went to grade school together. We faced some racism from other kids since my grade school was mostly Caucasian people but I generally got along with everyone. I managed to get straight A's all through grade school, but I also got into some minor fights which lead to a few trips to the principals office.

My first introduction to a barbell was when I was 14, and I learned how to do a shoulder press and a bicep curl. A good friend of our family was training for wrestling in high school, and he also showed me how to do some different types of push ups. I was currently training in tae kwon do and obtained a senior rank (red belt) before quitting to pursue bodybuilding.

As a young child, my parents noticed how much energy I had compared to my sisters. My parents put me into every sport they could think of, and I excelled in soccer, martial arts, and gymnastics. I found out quickly my talents did not lie in hockey, basketball, or baseball. I also noticed my head was bigger than the average kid, so my parents were happy when I started to lift weights. They figured if my muscles grew bigger it would balance out my bigger head.

My first barbell set was purchased at a well-known retail store, and this consisted of a 100 lb weight set, Olympic straight bar, and two adjustable dumbbells. I started a training regimen at 16 in my parent's basement and used the piano bench to do my exercises. The piano bench was very unstable, so I bought a real bench press apparatus and more weights to lift heavier. After grunting and groaning for a year, I noticed some bumps were beginning to form over my body as this was newly formed muscle. My progress was very slow, and I was still skinny. I secretly wanted to look like those guys in the muscle magazines but had no idea of the chemicals they were using. I attributed these slow gains to the lack of knowledge when it came to a very important component, the eating.

In grade 9, I had a crush on one of my sister's friends and one summer day we all went swimming, and she commented on how skinny I looked. My best friend at that time also worked out but had a better physique than me, which resulted in him meeting more girls every time we went out. One of the most defining moments of my life is when he set up a street fight with another guy since he had seen me spar in taekwondo. The plan backfired, and I ended up losing the fight. I knew how to fight, but I held back for some reason. After that, I decided not to hold back anymore and vowed to be a big, powerful, and respected person one day. What I wished for did come true but I suffered some serious consequences from allowing that to happen.

After researching, I eventually found a really good book on how to put on muscle naturally by eating. I finally realized the one secret to growth is to eat enough calories from food and supplements.

When grade 9 finished, my whole summer plan was to follow this new diet I'd created for myself and to really push myself with some heavy resistance training. For the whole summer, I did nothing but work out and I ate a tremendous amount of calories. In three months, my body weight jumped up from 150 lbs to 175 lbs. My diet consisted of meat sandwiches, cookies, milk, fruit, vegetables, and weight gain shakes. I also ate whatever my mom cooked as my caloric intake hit close to 4000 calories. Another thing that increased was the amount of times I had to go to the washroom. Thankfully, toilet paper is cheap. On top of that, my room started to smell like methane gas from all the protein farts. People who are reading this and eat a fair amount of protein can relate to this. All my clothes started to feel tight, and I looked and felt like a new human being, so in the end, it was all worth it.

When I went back to high school for grade 10, my new physique was a hit. People were staring at me, girls were really noticing me, and I was getting more respect from everyone. One girl even commented on how much attention I was going to get this year. The funny thing is, I eventually ended up dating the girl who gave me the comment. No more skinny Paul and I loved the new physique and identity.

In grade 11, my best friend and I made a decision to switch high schools. This eventually led to doing my first cycle in grade 12. This really muscular guy used to come around on our lunch breaks, and one day, I asked him how he got so big. After conversing about eating and training, he mentioned the use of anabolic steroids since he was preparing for a bodybuilding show. After researching about anabolic steroids, I made a decision to buy a bottle of testosterone from him. The bottle cost me $110 and was called testosterone cypionate. I would inject myself with 1 cc on Monday and 1 cc on Friday for the duration of 4 weeks. Then the last 2 weeks I would do 1 cc on Wednesday. This would give me 500 mg of testosterone a week and the last 2 weeks would be 250 mg. When I did get the bottle, the top cap was not on the bottle, and to this day I know it was only half strength. I did my first shot on the top of the quadriceps area with no problem. Some people have a hard time with needles, but the pain never bothered me. I just wanted to be big. My strength went up in the gym, and I started to eat more calories. My body weight went up to 181 lbs which is a 6 lb gain in 6 weeks. Not exactly Mr. Olympia material but I was happy to gain 6 lbs as I did not know what to expect.

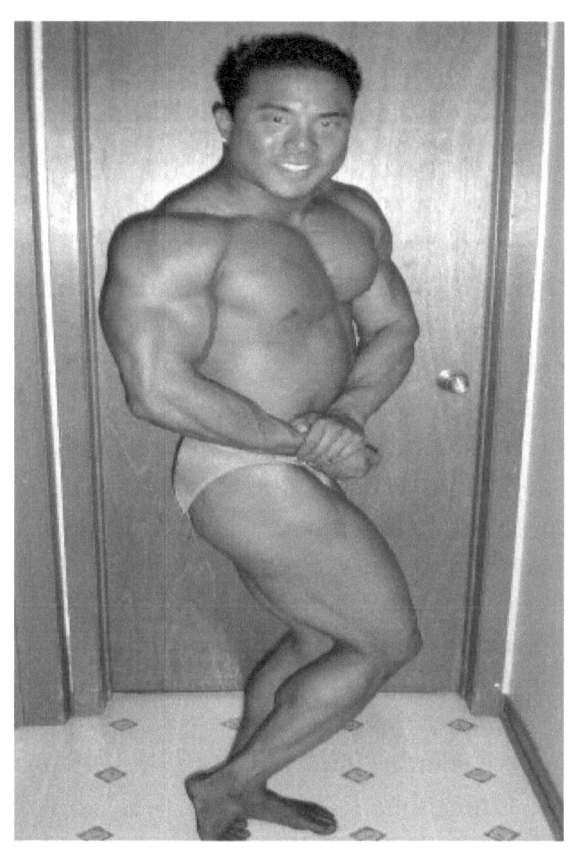

Side chest pose. Competition weight of 181 lbs. A few days after a level 3 show.

COMPETITION LIFESTYLE

Even though I had already qualified for level 2, my plan was to compete in a few more competitions in order to understand how my body reacted with everything. I was hooked on the competition lifestyle since I had already won a show. People who compete can relate to being addicted to the competition lifestyle. I competed a few more times and placed second and third before my plan was to get ready for a level 2 show. Once a person has worked so hard to achieve a certain look, it is hard to go back to looking normal. Looking like a freak is addictive as only ten percent of the human population can achieve this look.

Eating bland food like steamed broccoli and baked chicken breasts with no seasoning was becoming easier to do, and I started to use more steroids. One thing I always did was learn how to come off steroids properly, and this is why I am still healthy today. The coming off period to any steroid cycle is the least favourite part but is crucial to let a person's system rebalance itself. Everyone who cycles off will lose some muscle mass, but the goal of post cycle therapy is to minimize muscle loss and to restart the natural testosterone production process. I will get into more about post cycle therapy in the upcoming chapters.

Having a low percentage of body fat to show off the abdominals in the summer was one of the easiest ways to meet girls. From birth to age 17, I grew up in a church environment and was taught not to have sex before marriage. Even at church, I was always chasing girls around, but I did not become sexually active until later on in my life. I was a shy and nerdy kid growing up, but bodybuilding and testosterone changed all of that. Bodybuilding gave me more confidence with my looks and body, but the extra testosterone changed me into a raging hormone. With my new physique, girls would come up to me at the club, gym, beach, or at any public place. During a break from my one show, I was resting at Toronto Beaches with my shirt off. I was approached by two females, and they were curious to see if I carried a license for my chest. If my head was normal, I would have asked for their phone numbers, but all that was registering in my head was to drink water and to eat a hamburger. I then realized that male bodybuilders have to do less work when it comes to meeting females. This doesn't mean that every guy who weight trains and builds a physique will have similar results. Girls will often look at a guy's shoes, income level, clothes, hair, face, and personality.

As I increased my testosterone dosage, so did my sex drive. I started to turn into a sex maniac, and all I could think about was girls and sex. Most straight guys think about sex and girls all the time also, but this was different. It was like driving a car and never running out of gas. If I saw any girl bending over to tie her shoe, all I could think about was mounting her from behind. I started to have more sex with girls at clubs, girls from escort agencies, and girls who were considered my friends. Having sex with girls who were considered my friends brought me the most headaches as it never ended well. Having a great sex drive makes any guy feel good about themselves. When a guy stays on testosterone for a year and does not cycle off properly, he is shutting down his own natural testosterone supply. I will expand on that more in the upcoming chapter.

Being extremely built brought me some different type of work. I managed to work at some different jobs like doing security work at various night clubs across Niagara. At 5'8', I hovered between 190 lbs and 205 lbs. My boxing, wrestling, and tae kwon do background came in handy when our security team had to break up fights and toss people out of clubs. After seeing an ad for modelling in the newspaper, I decided to try out my looks and physique in the world of acting and modelling. Participants were to meet at a hotel auditorium, and various agents were there to view the people who were trying out. One by one we were called to the front, and all we had to say was our name and age. Almost every agent wanted to sign me up, so at that point I was pretty ecstatic. Next came the part where I was to talk to the agents who were interested in me and then I would make a decision who to work with. One agent said I looked like Bruce Lee, and if I did martial arts that would be perfect. I often wondered if he thought I owned a convenience store and ate with chop sticks. From there on, my work as an actor and model started to take off as I got various work for movies, television commercials, and a few photo shoots. This type of work would be only part-time because people who try to become a full-time actor always struggle to find more work. I soon lost interest in television when my agent asked if I was comfortable doing auditions where I would have to take my shirt off and kiss guys. I still have an agent, and to this day I don't mind doing an audition every once in a while, but as long as it fits into my current schedule.

Eating, training, steroids, and sleeping is the life of most competitive hard-core bodybuilders. Most bodybuilders and physique athletes become trainers or choose a low impact energy job as this fits into their lifestyle. When I was trying to climb up the competition ladder, I owned a nutrition store as that gave me the flexibility to eat and train at full capacity. Through the competitions, I became more regimented with my lifestyle when it came to eating, training, and sleeping. Even when travelling, my suitcase consisted of my clothes, steroids, and supplements. Before going to any place, I would check to see if the gym and food would be suitable for my bodybuilding needs.

Throughout my life, I understood the science behind the drugs, supplements, food, and the mindset of what it took to compete in bodybuilding. My friends and family always came to me for advice whether it would be about training, nutrition, or steroids. After winning my first show, I started to train people part-time and found it to be a rewarding job. For my first client, I ended pushing too hard at his first few sessions, but that is a mistake most trainers make when they first start. My first job I really enjoyed was at a nutrition store in downtown St. Catherine's. I quickly learned about the supplement industry and then went on to open my own nutrition store a few years after.

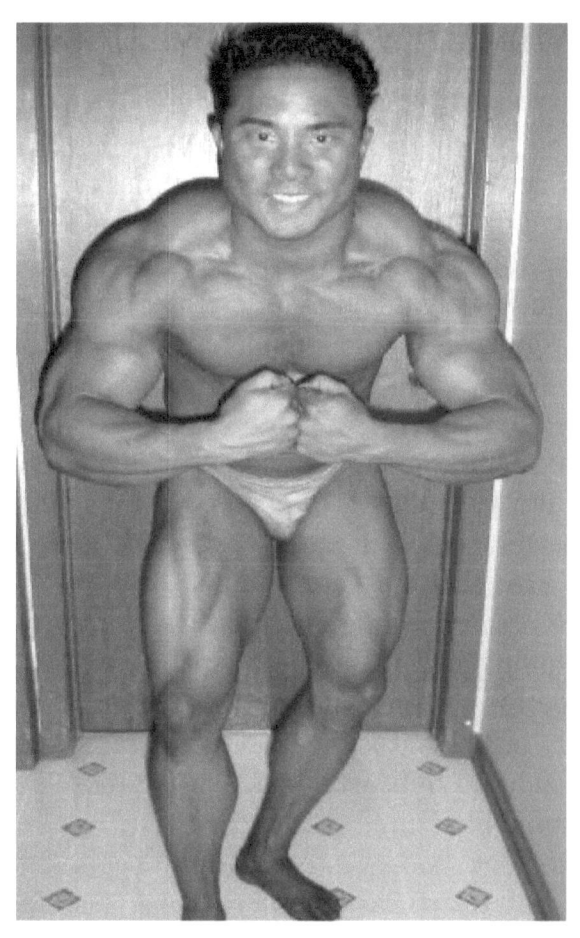

Most muscular pose. Competition weight of 181 lbs.
A few days after a level 3 show.

WHAT IT WOULD HAVE TAKEN TO TURN PRO

Now I continue the story from my first competition. After being at a low body weight for my first show, the first thing I wanted to do now was to gain back some body weight and muscle. After drinking fluids and gorging on food, a competitor can gain back up to 10 lbs in a few days. When a person finishes a competition, there is a window period where they can eat literally anything and not gain any body fat. Since the body has been starved for 10-12 weeks, the metabolism is fired up beyond normal, and all those extra calories are shuttled into the skeletal muscle or burned off. The trick is to know when to start eating clean again as some people end up eating garbage for a month and put on excessive amounts of body fat. This was the favourite part of competing as I would do light workouts and the muscle pumps were mind blowing.

The junk food festival would begin after the show was over. Pasta for breakfast, fast food for lunch, and then pizza for supper. Snacks would consist of chips, ice cream, and cookies. After eating like this for a few days, I would feel sick and then go back to my regular diet of eating clean. To add more size back on, I would eat clean carbohydrates such as brown rice, yams, and whole wheat pasta.

Next came the fun part, coming off my steroids to restore my testosterone levels and receptor sites. My rest period would be two months and then I would be on another cycle for three months.

Bodybuilders and physique athletes who compete generally have two stages. An offseason stage and competition stage. Sports athletes have different stages that they train for which is called periodization. During an offseason for a bodybuilder, the main goal is to put on muscle and to bring up any weak areas. So any serious competitor will have to assess their weak areas and try to bring them up to par with the stronger areas. For me, my problem area was always my upper back thickness. So my off season training was always structured towards bringing up my upper back thickness. My strongest areas were my hamstrings, quadriceps, and calves. This did not mean I would train them equally as hard, but they just grew faster than all my other body parts.

During the offseason and bulking stage, I used steroids that would give me the best mass gains. To put on the most size possible, I used a long- acting testosterone such as cypionate or ethanate. Some cycles would consist of Sustanon 250 as an alternative as this was a blend of four kinds of different testosterone. Next were the oral pills such as Dianabol or Anadrol. I would always stack one of these pills with the testosterone to maximize the muscle building effects. Anadrol is one of the strongest oral steroids a person can take and is highly anabolic. On a cycle of Anadrol and testosterone cypionate, a user could see gains of 20-30lbs of body weight when used properly. Other factors that affect gaining muscle when a person is on a cycle are genetics, training, caloric intake, and sleep. Anadrol is a toxic steroid, so I only used it for 2-3 weeks at a dosage of 50 mg daily and then stopped.

On a simple but large cycle of testosterone ethanate, Dianabol, and growth hormone, my body weight went up to 205 lbs. After level 1, I often threw in a few cycles of growth hormone a year to maximize more quality muscle growth. At 205 lbs, my arms measured 18.8 inches, neck measured 18.3 inches, and calves measured 18.4 inches at a height of 5'8'. These measurements were done when the muscles were cold so when pumped, my arms and calves would have been over 19 inches. The arms, calves, and neck of a good symmetrical bodybuilder should roughly be all the same size.

At a body weight of 205 lbs, I could lift tremendous amounts of weight. My incline bench press was 375 lbs for 2 repetitions, back squat was 405 lbs for 3 repetitions, and deadlift was 405 lbs for 2 repetitions. My eyes would go bloodshot after deadlifting and before doing back squats, my gym partner would slap my head to increase the adrenaline. People would look at me like I was some kind of freak and I loved it. My sisters did not approve of the new look and thought I looked gross. After successfully building up my upper back, it was so thick and full of muscle I fell down the stairs one day and got up like nothing happened. Luckily there were no injuries as my back muscles cushioned my fall.

The amount of calories I had to ingest in order to achieve 205 lbs was no easy task. My metabolism was very fast, so I had to consistently eat every two hours to gain muscle. My caloric intake reached over 5000 calories a day, and I was no stranger to the washroom. To consistently eat 5000 calories a day was like a chore but it had to be done. My day and activities all evolved four things: training, eating, steroids, and sleeping. Luckily I had a supplement store so my schedule was flexible as most people with normal jobs could not adhere to this type of schedule.

For breakfast, I would eat two cups of oatmeal, one serving of fruit, one cup of milk, and two scoops of protein powder. The majority of the calories came from lunch and dinner as I would usually eat fast food to get all those much-needed calories. A well-known fast food place served a double cheeseburger, large poutine fries, and an extra-large milkshake as a combo. This combo became my favourite lunch or dinner but not all the time. I would sometimes eat at my parents' house and a meal there would consist of two to three breaded chicken breasts, two to three cups of brown rice, and two cups of vegetables with dip. My snacks in between my meals would consist of a meal replacement shake which consisted of 52 grams of protein, 40 grams of carbohydrates, and 20 grams of fats. Competitive bodybuilding has nothing to do with health, and the goal is to be bigger and better in the next competition. The bulking phase is all about getting the required amount of calories for growth.

During the competition stage, the goal is to keep most of the muscle a person has gained during the offseason training. If my weight was 205 lbs, I would want to lose 15-20 lbs of body fat and then drop 10 lbs of water. My final competition weight would be 175 lbs, and this would put me on the top of the middleweight class. A gain of 21 lbs of muscle from my first competition.

My steroid cycle did change as the goal would be to lose body fat and maintain my current muscle mass. There would be no break from the offseason cycle to the competition cycle as taking a break would result in losing muscle mass. The length of my competition cycles was 10 weeks long as this gave me sufficient time to make the required changes. For the first 4 weeks, I would use Sustanon 250, Decca Durabolin, clenbuterol, and growth hormone. The last 5 weeks I would use testosterone propionate, trenbolone, Winstrol, clenbuterol, Cytomel, and growth hormone. The last 2 weeks I would stop the testosterone propionate and growth hormone. For the last 2 weeks, I would use

Arimidex and the last week would be haladrol and diuretics. My body was a chemical pool of performance enhancing drugs, but the end result was a freaky looking human being.

As I increased my dosages, the side effects became more apparent. Two things I really noticed was a big change in my temper and my way of thinking. Road rage was becoming normal to me, and this was not a good thing. One day I was driving, and a guy gave me the middle finger, so I got out of the car and tried to open his car door in the middle of the road. Luck was on his side as the door was locked. To this day, I am glad his door was locked as I would have beaten him senseless. A few of my girlfriends mentioned I did say weird things to them during my last few weeks of competition. I attribute this to the lack of calories, intense training, and all the chemicals that were inside of my body. Any drug when taken over a long period of time can change the way a person acts and thinks.

During my 5-6 years of heavy steroid use, I only went to the hospital once. My leg got infected by a shot I did in my side quadriceps before a level 3 show. Like an idiot, I still competed, but in reality, a trip to the hospital would have been the smarter move. After the show was over, my sisters drove me to the hospital because my leg could not bend fully. The doctor gave me some antibiotics and told me that if the infection had gone to my blood stream, I could have died. My mentality back then was to be big and to die being big.

During my last try at the OBBA provincials (level 3), I had managed to get third place in the middleweight class out of nine guys. Top 3 would advance to the nationals, and I would have a year to prepare for the nationals. Once again, I would have to re-assess my weak areas, drug regimen, and nutritional intake in order to bring my physique to the next level. The OBBA federation existed before the OPA federation and required the athlete to compete at four different levels before turning professional. A competitor had to be placed in top 3 in all three levels and then win their class at the nationals in order to achieve professional status.

To add more size to my physique, I started to use insulin. Insulin is a powerful hormone that is made by the pancreas and controls the level of sugar glucose in the human body. The idea behind insulin use is to shuttle more amino acids and glucose into the muscle cells creating muscle protein synthesis. This is one serious drug that can kill a person when used improperly. I only used insulin in the offseason as it was easier to control because my caloric intake was high. This is a drug a person does not want to stay on for a year as they would become type 1 diabetic. I only used insulin for four weeks as becoming diabetic was not on my agenda. One famous professional bodybuilder I knew used to inject himself with over 100 units a week. Using 100 units a week is equivalent to a bottle of insulin. He eventually became type 1 diabetic and weighed close to 270 lbs of pure muscle. He is dead now.

After using growth hormone for a few years, I started to see some of the side effects on my body. Other than the mind blowing muscle pumps, my jawline and elbows started to grow also. This was not a good thing as my modelling and acting required my face to look normal. After stopping the growth hormone, my jaw and elbow returned back to normal size, but it took a few months.

From 19-24, I competed in over 12 bodybuilding shows and started to feel the side effects from all the drugs, physically and physiologically. I was addicted to my physique and to being chemically enhanced. My family, friends, and doctor started to worry about my health, and getting nose bleeds from high blood pressure was becoming a normal thing to me. I started to wonder if all of this was worth it. Bodybuilders have to spend thousands of dollars to get ready for a show, and all they get in return is a trophy and some health issues.

When the competition date for the Nationals was announced, I got some mixed feelings about competing in Calgary. To achieve professional status would mean going well over 1000 mg of testosterone and doubling all my current dosages of steroids. If I did continue to compete, my health would be compromised, and that was a route I was not willing to take. In the end, I decided to not compete in the OBBA federation anymore but decided to pursue another venture, mixed martial arts.

CHEMICALLY ENHANCED - MY DIET AND TRAINING DURING OFF SEASON

Here is an example of my eating plan when I was in a bulking phase. This is the exact diet for day 1 when my body weight was 205 lbs and bench pressing 375 lbs. My goal was to be as big as possible but never to go over 1000 mg of testosterone. You will notice the lack of vegetables and excessive amounts of fast food. I have included the caloric intake to show the total amount consumed.

Meal 1 - 8:00am
2 cups of oatmeal
1 serving fruit
2 cups of whey protein
1 cup 2 % milk
1 vita C 500 mg
723 calories

Snack 1 - 10:00 am
1 package meal replacement powder
400 calories

Meal 3 - 12:00 pm
3 bacon cheeseburgers
1 large French fries with ketchup

1 large chocolate milkshake
1560 calories

Snack 2 - 2:00 pm
1 package meal replacement powder
400 calories

Snack 3 - 4:00 pm
1 package meal replacement powder
400 calories

Meal 4 - 6:00 pm
1 double whopper
1 large poutine
1 large strawberry milkshake
1630 calories

Meal 5 - 9:00 pm
8-ounce chicken breast with barbecue sauce
1 cup brown rice
1 cup vegetables with ranch dip
472 calories

Total caloric intake - 5586 calories

TRAINING SCHEDULE

This is a week's schedule of what my training looked like when I was 205 lbs. This would be a low repetition and a heavy week. My non-active days were on Wednesday and Saturday. I would pyramid upwards with more weight for each set and would use 90 % of my 1 rep max for my last set. The only type of cardio I would do was light walking as my focus was more geared towards resistance training.

Sunday: Light walking for 25-30 minutes
Monday: Back + hamstrings + core
Tuesday: Chest + shoulders
Wednesday: Rest
Thursday: Quadriceps + calves + traps
Friday: Triceps + biceps + forearms + core
Saturday: Rest

MONDAY

Back
1. Dead lifts - 1x10, 1x8, 1x6, 1x4, 1x2 reps
2. Chin ups - 1x10, 1x8, 1x6, 1x4, 1x2 reps
3. Barbell back rows - 1x10, 1x8, 1x6, 1x4, 1x2 reps
4. Seated back pulley rows - 1x10, 1x8, 1x6, 1x4, 1x2 reps

5. Under grip chin-ups - 1x10, 1x8, 1x6, 1x4 reps

Hamstrings
1. Machine lying leg curls - 1x10, 1x8, 1x6, 1x4, 1x2 reps
2. Standing leg curls - 1x10, 1x8, 1x6, 1x4, 1x2 reps

Core
1. Bench v-ups - 1x30,1x30,1x30 reps
2. Standing bar twists - 2 x 1 minute

TUESDAY

Chest
1. Flat bench press - 1x10, 1x8, 1x6, 1x4, 1x2 reps
2. Incline bench press - 1x10, 1x8, 1x6, 1x4, 1x2 reps
3. Flat dumbbell fly - 1x10, 1x8, 1x6, 1x4 reps
4. Incline dumbbell fly - 1x10, 1x8, 1x6, 1x4 reps

Shoulders
1. Dumbbell seated press - 1x10, 1x8, 1x6, 1x4, reps
2. Dumbbell side laterals - 1x10, 1x8, 1x6, 1x4 reps
3. Straight bar upright rows - 1x10, 1x8, 1x6, 1x4 reps
4. Dumbbell bent over laterals - 1x10, 1x8, 1x6, 1x4 reps

THURSDAY

Quadriceps
1. Plate loader leg press - 1x10, 1x8, 1x6, 1x4, 1x2 reps
2. Barbell back squats - 1x10, 1x8, 1x6, 1x4, 1x2 reps
3. Leg extensions - 1 x10, 1x8, 1x6, 1x4, 1x2 reps
4. Hack squats - 1 x10, 1x8, 1x6, 1x4, 1x2 reps

Calves
1. Seated calf raises - 1x20, 1x15, 1x12, 1x10, 1x8 reps
2. Standing calf raises - 1x20, 1x15, 1x12, 1x10, 1x8 reps

Traps
1. Barbell front shrugs - 1x10, 1x8, 1x6, 1x4, 1x2 reps

FRIDAY

Triceps
1. Pulley push downs - 1x10, 1x8, 1x6, 1x4 reps
2. W-bar skull crushers - 1x10, 1x8, 1x6, 1x4 reps
3. Pulley rope overhead extensions - 1x10, 1x8, 1x6, 1x4 reps

Biceps

1. Barbell bicep curls - 1x10, 1x8, 1x6, 1x4 reps
2. Incline dumbbell curls - 1x10, 1x8, 1x6, 1x4 reps
3. One arm cable concentration curls - 1x10, 1x8, 1x6 reps

Forearms
1. Partial reverse preacher curls - 1x12, 1x10, 1x8 reps
2. Behind the body bar curls - 1x12, 1x10, 1x8 reps

Core
1. Bird dogs - 2x20 reps
2. Incline leg raises - 3x25 reps
3. Incline sit ups - 3x25 reps
5. Dumbbell side tilts - 2x15 each side

COMING OFF AND MAINTAINING

The period when a person comes off their cycle is called Post Cycle Therapy (PTC). The purpose is to kick-start a person's natural testosterone production and to help maintain muscle mass throughout the transition. When a person uses anabolic steroids, they suppress their own natural testosterone production.

Men produce testosterone in their testicles. For men to produce testosterone, the pituitary must release a hormone called Luteinizing hormone (LH) and Follicle stimulating hormone (FHS). When a person uses testosterone or steroids, this tells the pituitary gland to produce less LH and FSH which results in less testosterone production. When the person stops using steroids, the person is still producing less testosterone, and with PCT use, the goal is to help kick start the natural testosterone production again.

Coming down from 205 lbs to 175 lbs and then maintaining a physique I felt comfortable with was not an easy thing to do. My old clothes no longer fit properly, and I lost roughly 20-30 percent of my strength in the gym. Seeing myself regress was not an easy thing to do, but it had to be done in order to be healthy again.

Any bodybuilder or athlete that cares about their health knows that coming off is important to protect their hormonal balance. Proper planning is required in order to maintain their muscle mass and to support the body throughout the transition period.

My list of PCT drugs to help me come off my cycle was Clomid, Arimidex, and Human Chorionic Gonadotropin (HCG). Arimidex was used to stop any excessive estrogen conversion from happening. To stop testicular shrinkage or make them grow back, I used HCG. Clomid would be used to increase the Luteinizing hormone (LH), so more testosterone would be produced. By combining all three of these together, at the end of my cycle, this would help my body to produce more testosterone levels naturally.

On top of the PCT drugs, I also used supplements such as creatine tri-malate, arginine, fat burners, and testosterone boosters. When a person comes off steroids, this will result in a loss of blood volume, muscle mass and decreased nitrogen retention. The creatine tri-malte did help to keep my muscles full of water and keep my strength up. I used arginine for its vasodilation abilities, as well as its ability to participate in protein synthesis. The testosterone boosters would be used after the Clomid to keep my natural testosterone levels up. I always used protein powder, glutamine, and vitamins whether I was on cycle or not.

A person who loses muscle mass will also lose strength. Loss of muscle mass will result in a slower basal metabolic rate (BMR). The BMR is defined as the amount of energy expended while at rest in the post-absorptive state. All these factors must be considered when a person plans their off cycle training and eating. My strength dropped drastically even with the help of creatine, arginine, and testosterone boosters. I could still bench 275 lbs for 2 repetitions, deadlift 315 for 2 repetitions, and back squat 315 for 4 repetitions. As my physique started to change, I noticed how sore my muscles were at first and this resulted in a longer rest period in between training days. My training schedule had to be changed because I was no longer chemically enhanced. I have included two training schedules that show the difference in training frequency when chemically enhanced versus being natural.

As stated earlier, when a person loses 10-20 lbs of muscle, their basal metabolic rate slows down. This affects a person's rate of digestion and absorption of food and nutrients. If I continued to eat over 5000 calories a day post cycle, I would be really obese. Instead of getting auditions for a lean fit Asian guy, I would get auditions for a fat Asian guy. My diet would no longer consist of fast food but more healthy choices from carbohydrates, proteins, and good fats. I would still eat like a bodybuilder and follow the same meal structure but just less quantity. An example of one of my meals during my transition phase would be two cups of pasta with sauce, two barbecue chicken breasts, and two cups of steamed broccoli. My caloric intake would be above 3000 calories, and this would be sufficient to maintain my natural physique.

Buying new clothes was not a chore to me but going down a few sizes was not a fun thing to do. I grew up with two older sisters, so shopping was a normal thing to me. Getting used to my new shell and body weight of 175 lbs was one of the toughest transitions, both mentally and physically. My plan was to try and stay natural in order to clean out my system and become a healthy person again. Seeing my muscles shrink and then having some of my old friends commenting how much size I lost did not help the situation. My pumps in the gym were nothing like before. No more mind blistering pumps from the chemicals but just normal muscle pumps.

Some men can develop a condition called muscle dysmorphia. This is a condition where the person is obsessed with thinking that their body is too small, insufficiently muscular, or insufficiently lean. In most conditions, the person's build is above average. Understanding this condition helped me mentally to understand that my mind was not in tune with my body as I often felt my physique was never good enough.

I have always have been strong mentally but coming off any drug and staying off is not always an easy thing to accomplish. People always struggle with some type of addiction whether it is food, alcohol, caffeine, or a certain type of behaviour. In order to come off steroids, a person must be ready and have a plan in place. When the risks outweigh the rewards, that is usually a good indicator to stop.

NATURAL STATE - MY DIET AND TRAINING DURING THE OFF SEASON

This is a good example of my diet when I was in a bulking phase. I would set a goal to gain 10 lbs in two months, and I would let my body fat percentage go over ten percent. A cheat meal would be incorporated every third day, and that would consist either a half a plate of meat lasagne, two cheeseburgers, or two to three slices of pizza. You will notice a much more balanced diet of fruits, vegetables, proteins, and carbohydrates in comparison to the previous bulking diet.

Meal 1 - 5:30 am
1 cup steel cut oats
1 scoop whey protein powder
1 cup water
500 mg vitamin C
2000 units vitamin D
2 omega 3 capsules

Meal 2 - 8:00 am
2 whole eggs with ketchup and cheese
1 cup raw kale
1 medium size banana
2 slices flax bread with 2 tsp natural peanut butter

Snack 1 - 10:00 am
1 scoop   whey powder
1/2 cup   steel cut oats
1 cup water

Meal 3 - 12:00 pm
8oz lean ground   turkey with barbecue sauce
2 cups of cucumber and carrots with balsamic vinegar
2 cup cooked pasta with 1 cup spaghetti sauce

Snack 2 - 3:00 pm
1 scoop   whey powder
1/2 cup   steel cut oats
1 cup water

Meal 4 - 6:00 pm
8 oz pork tenderloin with garlic, salt, pepper
2 cups brown rice
2-3 cups of raw lettuce and spinach with Caesar dressing

Snack 3 - 8:30 pm
6-7 oz chicken leg with curry sauce
1 cup natural yogurt
1 scoop   whey protein

TRAINING SCHEDULE

This is what my training schedule looks like when I want to put on muscle and bulk up. One big difference is the amount of rest I give myself after a resistance training session. When a person is natural, they take longer to recover as resistance training tears apart the muscle fibers. My cardiovascular workouts only consisted of 20-25 minutes as this is just to keep my VO2 levels up. This would be a low repetition and a heavy week. I would pyramid upwards with more weight for each set and would use 90 % of my 1 rep max for my last set.

Sunday: Back + hamstrings + traps
Monday: Rest
Tuesday: Cardio + core
Wednesday: Quadriceps + chest + forearms
Thursday: Rest
Friday: Cardio + core
Saturday: Shoulders + triceps + biceps + calves

SUNDAY

Back
1. Chin ups - 1x10, 1x8, 1x6, 1x4, 1x2 reps

2. Under grip pull downs - 1x10, 1x8, 1x6, 1x4, 1x2 reps
3. Barbell back rows - 1x10, 1x8, 1x6, 1x4, 1x2 reps
4. Seated pulley rows - 1x10, 1x8, 1x6, 1x4, 1x2 reps

Hamstrings
1. Lying leg curls - 1x10, 1x8, 1x6, 1x4 reps
2. Stiff legged hamstrings - 1x10, 1x8, 1x6, 1x4 reps

Traps
1. Barbell front shrugs - 1x10, 1x8, 1x6, 1x4 reps

TUESDAY

Cardio
1. Bike - 10 minutes
2. Tread mile - 15 minutes

Core
1. Stability ball reverse hyperextension - 3x20 reps
2. Stability ball passes - 3x20 reps
4. Side planks - 1x1 minute each side

WEDNESDAY

Quadriceps
1. Leg extensions - 1x10, 1x8, 1x6, 1x4, 1x2 reps
2. Back squats - 1x10, 1x8, 1x6, 1x4, 1x2 reps

3. Plate loader leg press - 1x10, 1x8, 1x6, 1x4, 1x2 reps
4. Holding dumbbell lunges - 1x10, 1x8, 1x6, 1x4 reps

Chest
1. Decline bench press - 1x10, 1x8, 1x6, 1x4 reps
2. Incline bench press - 1x10, 1x8, 1x6, 1x4 reps
3. Flat dumbbell fly - 1x10, 1x8, 1x6, 1x4 reps
4. Incline dumbbell fly - 1x10, 1x8, 1x6, 1x4 reps

Forearms
1. Dumbbell hammer curls - 1x12, 1x10, 1x8 reps
2. Seated bench flexor curls - 1x12, 1x10, 1x8 reps

FRIDAY

Cardio
1. Machine rowing - 10 minutes
2. Elliptical - 15 minutes

Core
1. Holding dumbbell good mornings - 3x20 reps
2. Reverse crunches - 3x20 reps
3. Cable crunches - 3x20 reps
4. Pulley twists - 2x20 reps each side

SATURDAY

Shoulders
1. Machine press - 1x10, 1x8, 1x6, 1x4 reps
2. Dumbbell side laterals - 1x10, 1x8, 1x6, 1x4 reps
3. Front seated barbell press - 1x10, 1x8, 1x6, 1x4 reps
4. Machine rear laterals - 1x10, 1x8, 1x6, 1x4 reps

Triceps
1. Pulley bar push downs - 1x10, 1x8, 1x6, 1x4 reps
2. Close grip bench press - 1x10, 1x8, 1x6, 1x4 reps
3. Dumbbell overhead extensions - 1 x10, 1x8, 1x6, 1x4 reps

Biceps
1. Alternate dumbbell curls - 1x10, 1x8, 1x6, 1x4 reps
2. Pulley overhead curls - 1x10, 1x8, 1x6 reps
3. One arm preacher dumbbell curls - 1x10, 1x8, 1x6 reps

Calves
1. Plate loader leg press, calf raises - 1x20, 1x15, 1x12, 1x10, 1x8 reps
2. Seated calf raises - 1x20, 1x15, 1x12, 1x10, 1x8 reps

BEING SMART ABOUT DOSAGES AND HEALTH

Steroids and other performance-enhancing drugs are often easily accessible through the street, website, or doctors. Some are made in labs, but most are made in underground labs. Different countries have different laws pertaining to steroids and various other performance enhancing drugs, so it is always best to know the laws before purchasing these drugs. Anyone who wants to enhance their performance in sports or just at the gym has used anabolic steroids at some point as they are easily accessible. Performance enhancing drugs are considered a grey area as even police officers are known to use steroids as seen in a well-known previous Mr. Olympian.

If I can give some advice on this topic, it would be about knowing the source, knowing your physical limitations, and having the proper knowledge of what you are putting inside your body. Be realistic with your genetics as everyone cannot look like a Mr. Olympian or a top fitness model. People often think that more is always better or they assume combining more steroids together will produce faster results. While this is true to some degree, using excessive amounts will always lead to greater side effects and long-term health problems. When putting together a cycle, educate yourself on the different properties of all the steroids as you do not want to mix drugs that have the same effect on the body. An example would be using Decca Durabolin and equipoise together in a cycle. They are both anabolic and possess the hardening abilities that are seen when combined with a testosterone like propionate. They both suppress testosterone levels in a person's body so using them together would have a very negative impact on a person's natural testosterone production. If a guy wants to know what it would be like to be a girl, then I would suggest he use that combination with no testosterone in a cycle. Knowing the proper combinations will save a person the embarrassment with these kinds of issues.

Another health concern while a person uses steroids is to watch their HDL and LDL cholesterol levels. Most steroids will decrease a person's good cholesterol (HDL) and increase their bad cholesterol (LDL). A build-up of LDL cholesterol can result in a heart attack or stroke. Taking an omega 3 supplement during a cycle is a good idea as omega 3 fatty acids have been shown to lower the LDL levels inside of the human body. Another thing a person can do is to eat more foods that contain more of these good fats such as flaxseed oil, fish oil, chia seeds, walnuts, fish roe (eggs), fatty fish, seafood, soybeans, and spinach. If a person is planning to cycle on and off for years, going to see the doctor once or twice a year for a check-up is recommended. A doctor can do blood work and check to see if a person's HDL and LDL levels are balanced with each other.

It is always a good idea to plan a steroid cycle and know what dosages are appropriate for your goals. Don't just buy something and hope for the best as this usually does not turn out well. If you have limited knowledge seek out some advice from a doctor, top level bodybuilder or even the internet, which has a few good sites. Testosterone Nation (T-Nation) is a fairly good site where people write articles about bodybuilding, training, supplements, and performance enhancing drugs. Just use your common sense when reading an article as everything is not accurate and true.

What was your last meal? My last meal consisted of steak and a Greek salad. We all know steak comes from a cow, so we know where the meat came from. The point I am making here is always know and trust your source. If you purchase Decca, make sure it is not fake or something else. I have heard countless stories of people getting ripped off and taking fake or bad steroids which usually results in no gains or a trip to the hospital. There is nothing worse than an athlete or bodybuilder getting ready for competition and getting fake or the wrong type of steroids. This is dangerous as the person does not know what they are injecting themselves with. The person who is selling the steroids should have above knowledge of the drugs and their products. Lastly, use common sense and be street smart. If something is too good to be true, it usually is.

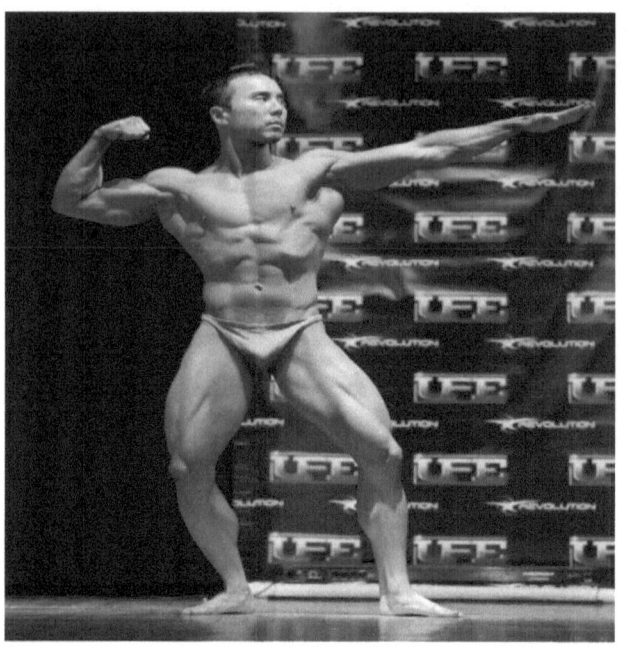

Competition weight of 168 lbs. A more natural body weight.

LIFE AFTER FORTY

As I am writing this update I am now 44 years of age. I was 38 when I wrote this book. When you read the conclusion remember it was written when I first published the book. This is an update on how my life has been going.

It has been 6 years since I started testosterone replacement therapy (TRT). My body weight is now 175 at 11% body fat at a height of 5'8'. I don't train as hard as I used because of my age and injuries, but I still enjoy a heavy resistance training session. I can still back squat 315 lbs for four reps, incline bench press 215 lbs for two reps, and do side laterals with 50 lbs for four reps.

After 40, you have to train differently. At the ages of 20 and 30, our bodies can handle more abuse. After 40, we want to take care extra care of our health. If we don't, we will have severe health issues at ages 50 and older.

What happens after the age of 40? Our testosterone and growth hormone levels drop by around one percent each year. Our testosterone levels actually start to decline in our 30s. This affects your muscle mass, bone mass, sex drive, energy levels, and immune system. Here is interesting information on how your testosterone levels affect our immune system.

Researchers from the Stanford School of Medicine published a study on testosterone and immunity, which found that men with higher levels of testosterone had a reduced response to the flu vaccine.

The study looked at the levels of antibodies in test subjects and compared each man's response to their testosterone levels. The study also found that women had a stronger antibody response to the flu vaccine than men, but that men with lower testosterone levels had a similar response to women.

Scientists are wondering if this may be linked to the fact that women often have stronger immune responses to viral, fungal, bacterial, and parasitic infections. Women also tend to have a stronger response to certain vaccines.

What is the underlining message of this research article? If you have high levels of testosterone or low levels of testosterone, your immune system may be negatively affected. You need to be in a normal range, which is between 300 and 1,000 nanograms per deciliter (ng/dL).

If you have lower testosterone and growth hormone levels, your recovery from exercise will take longer. Testosterone levels also affect protein synthesis. Most people know that muscle needs protein to help rebuild the torn muscle tissue from resistance training. Testosterone helps to decrease protein breakdown inside the body, so more can be utilized. This means you should need to rest longer in between your resistance training workouts and train at a lower intensity or volume after the age of 40.

Here is my schedule for how I now train. I have a suitable balance that works with my body when it comes to resistance training, cardio, and core. It is basically the same schedule as my natural state training. I train heavy one week using 80-90% of my 1RM, and then I switch to a lighter week using only 50-60% of my 1RM. This gives my joints a rest and stops me from over training. You will also notice I take at least two rest days. I also take more time off in between my resistance training days. On my heavy weeks, if I am not feeling fully recovered, I just skip a cardio and core day, which gives me an extra day of rest. Instead of doing cardio and core, I do five minutes of cardio as a warm up, five minutes of stretching, and then foam rolling for my entire body. Foam rolling is a great way to create more blood flow and enhance recovery.

EXAMPLE TRAINING WEEK

Sunday: Back + Shoulders + Traps
Monday: Rest
Tuesday: Cardio+Core
Wednesday: Chest + Quadriceps+ Calves
Thursday: Rest
Friday: Cardio+Core + Glutes
Saturday: Hamstrings+ Triceps + Biceps + Forearms
Sunday: Rest

TESTOSTERONE REPLACEMENT THERAPY DOSAGES

Always be smart about your dosages. It is best to start with a lower dosage and see how you respond to the testosterone. My dosages range from 60 to 80mg per shot. My dosage schedule is Monday and Thursday mornings, giving me between 120 and 160mg per week. I have gone up to 200mg per week but, I found I was adding too much muscle to my frame again. I have no desire to be 185 pounds again. Anything above 400mg is considered a bodybuilding dosage and will cause more severe side effects, as we learned earlier.

My preference for testosterone to use for TRT is cypionate or enanthate. The reason behind this is that both are long-acting esters, and they are easier to manage with the side effects. I have used all types of testosterone before and these two are my favourites for TRT. Testosterone cypionate has a half-life of eight days. Testosterone enanthate has a half-life of seven days. They are both similar, but I am currently using cypionate right now. I like to switch between the two every six months.

I like to do my shots in the afternoon, as that seems to work best for my body. Our levels of testosterone are highest in the morning and lowest at night. During the afternoon, my test levels start to drop, and by taking a shot in the afternoon, I get a small boost of energy. If I were to take testosterone at night, it may affect my sleeping patterns. Remember, everyone is different, so what works for my body may not work for your body. It is best to try in the morning and then in the afternoon and see what feels best for your system.

Do I feel any side effects from TRT? As you have learned earlier, excessive testosterone dosages can cause increased high blood pressure, increased aggression, and raging boners. The right dosage for your body can make you feel like you're 25 again. The key is to start with a low dosage and slowly increase your dosage. I also get yearly blood work. This is extremely important, as you want to see what your free and total testosterone levels are. Other things to check for are estradiol, prolactin, SHBG, and lipids. Another tool I found useful in keeping healthy while on TRT is to do blood donations every year.

An expected potential side effect of TRT is an increased level of red blood cells, which manifests as increased levels of hemoglobin and hematocrit. Your blood becomes thicker than normal. This "side effect" is actually a desired therapeutic effect in men with anemia but not a desired effect in normal men. How do you combat this unwanted side effect? Donate blood two to three times a year. I have been donating blood for four to five years, and this helps to keep my iron, hemoglobin, and hemocrit levels at a normal level.

Donating blood is a win-win situation. You get to save a life, reduce the risk of cardiovascular disease, and get a free blood analysis. What more could you ask for?

Blood viscosity is known to be a unifying factor in the risk for cardiovascular disease. How thick and sticky your blood is and how much friction your blood creates through the blood vessels can determine how much damage is done to the cells lining your arteries. You can reduce your blood viscosity by donating blood a few times a year, which eliminates the iron that may possibly oxidize in your blood. An increase in oxidative stress can be damaging to your cardiovascular system.

The removal of oxidative iron from the body through blood donations means less iron oxidation and reduced cardiovascular diseases.

I try to drink 10-12 glasses of water a day to combat the blood thickness caused by testosterone. A good general rule is to stay hydrated for general health and wellness. We all know the importance of water for bodily functions. It flushes out toxins, maximizes performance, maintains brain function, and does many other positive things in our body.

How does drinking extra water help with hemocrit levels? It is important to remember that hemoglobin is very dependent on your hydration levels. Dehydration causes the blood to become thicker. The combination of blood thickness with TRT is a recipe for disaster.

What you eat directly affects how you feel and respond on TRT. As you have learned earlier, after 40, we have to take extra care of our health. Another way to do this is to eat a well- balanced diet of protein, carbs, and fats. I still eat very healthy, but I like to indulge at lunch. My calorie count is around 2300-2800 every day. My diet now consists of raw vegetables three times a day and fruit two times a day. I limit sugar, processed foods, and certain types of fats. I also take an omega-3 fatty acid supplement for heart, brain, and cardiovascular health. One thing I noticed as we age is that we do not have to eat as much food. Our metabolism and digestion start to slow down naturally.

MY DIET ON TRT

Breakfast(shake) - 6:00am
1/2 scoop whey protein
1 raw egg
1cup kale
1 banana
1 omega 3 capsule

Shake 1 – 9:00am
3 1/4 cup oatmeal
1/2 scoop whey protein
1/2 cup fruit

Lunch – 11:30am
2 slices pepperoni pizza
2 cup veggies
3 tsp salad dressing
3oz chicken

Shake 2 – 2:00pm
3 1/4 cup oatmeal
1/2 scoop whey protein
1 tsp natural peanut butter

Supper – 5:00pm
7 oz pork
2 cups raw vegetables

Snack – 7:30pm
5 oz breaded chicken
1 cup plain yogurt

HEALTH IS WEALTH

Joe Rogan and Salvestor Stallone are a few celebrities who use testosterone replacement therapy. Every professional bodybuilder who is retired has to be on TRT. One of my friends, who recently turned 47 started on TRT. The first thing he noticed was more energy and increased mental clarity. I am not here to push hormone therapy or testosterone on anyone. My body actually needs it since I used testosterone when I was bodybuilding. If there is a hormone that helps you with anti- aging and you have the proper knowledge on how to use it, why not utilize it to its full potential?

Testosterone therapy is not a miracle drug that will magically cure your energy levels and libido. You must also weight train, eat healthy, take supplements, and follow certain protocols to feel the full effects.

Men who have prostate cancer or breast cancer are not suitable for testosterone therapy. Men who also have severe urinary tract problems, untreated severe sleep apnea, or uncontrolled heart failure should stay away from testosterone.

We already know the many benefits of weight training for our health. Another benefit weight training helps with is nitric oxide production. After 30, our nitric oxide levels also drop naturally by 20% every 10 years. Exercise really does get your blood pumping, largely because it improves endothelial function. Endothelium refers to the thin layer of cells that line the blood vessels. These cells produce nitric oxide, which keeps blood vessels healthy. Insufficient nitric oxide production results in endothelium dysfunction, which can contribute to atherosclerosis, high blood pressure, and other risk factors for heart disease.

Exercise keeps your endothelial cells and blood vessels healthy by increasing your body's natural ability to produce nitric oxide. Nitric oxide and testosterone go hand in hand because they both support sexual function in the male body.

The underlining message when we turn 40 is to take extra care of our bodies. We want to set up our long-term health for when we are 50 and older. Health is wealth. Always exercise, eat healthy, take supplements, and get a physical done at least once a year.

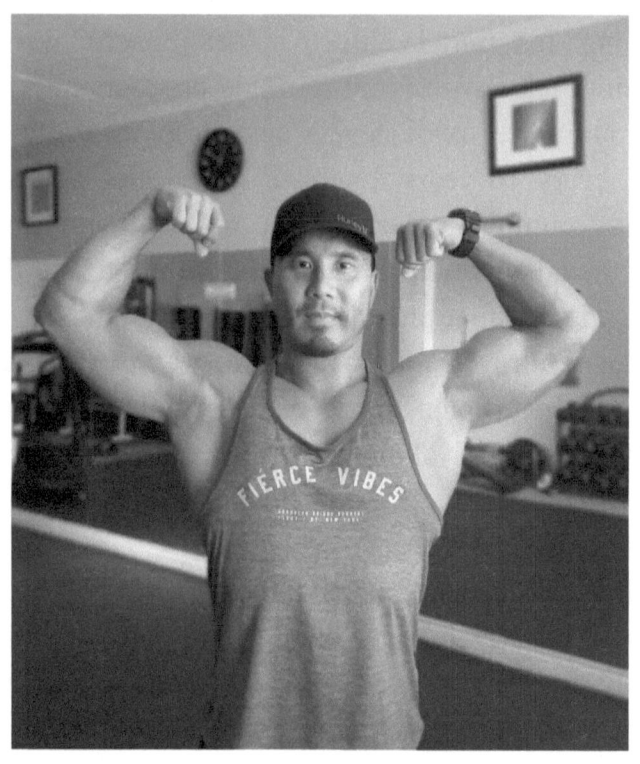

*A healthy body weight of 175lbs with 11% body fat
at the age of 44.*

STICKS AND STONES MAY BREAK MY BONES: I MISS BEING SKINNY

Here is a blog that I wrote about how I miss being skinny. I decided to include it at the end of my book.

Sticks. Bones. Twig. These are the names I remembered being called when I was a kid. Having braces, being smart, and playing the clarinet did not help with my self esteem issues. The good old days? I am thankful for having a good family but being skinny and getting picked on was not fun.

It seems like obesity is one of the biggest health concerns now in today's society. Let us not forget about the smaller percent of the population, the skinny people.

Here are four things I miss about being skinny:

1. Getting Very Little Attention From Girls
When your a twig, people don't notice you at all. Especially at the beach or a swimming pool. Muscle commands respect. When I was 205lbs of muscle, people use to stare at me like I was some kind of freak. I loved the attention. Was I healthy, no. Was I jacked on performance enhancing drugs, yes. The bottom line here is if you workout and keep in shape, people respect and notice you more.

2. Being Picked On

No one likes a bully. They are seen in everywhere in school and even in politics. When your skinny, you get picked on. I use to get picked on in grade school all the time. All that changed when I started to get serious about weight lifting in grade 10. After putting on 20lbs of muscle and some fat, no one bothered me anymore. The only drawback was all the food I had to eat and the extra trips to the washroom. When you exercise it helps to boost your self confidence and mood. Who knows, that bully may even stop bothering you at work.

3. Looking Funny In Clothes

When your skinny, even the tightest jeans don't fit properly. If your built from doing all those squats, your legs and butt will look perfect in those jeans. People judge each other on what type of clothes they wear and how they fit. I use to dress like a hip hop artist in grade 9. Baggy jeans, baggy shirt, and a hat backwards. I looked like an Asian homey. That lasted for a year until I started to realize I wasn't cool. After putting on 20 lbs of muscle and dressing like a normal human being, I started to get the respect I was looking for. How you look and dress will affect how people perceive you.

4. People Automatically Think Your Sick

Are you feeling okay? Did you eat enough today? Those are the questions I use to get in grade school. When your a twig, people think your undernourished or have some sort of disease. This is true to some degree as sick people have a hard time eating and are underweight. When your buff or fit, you exude confidence and health. What do you eat? How often do you workout? These are the types of questions I get now.

CONCLUSION

As I am writing this book, I am completely natural and my supplements today consist of protein powder, vitamins, testosterone boosters, and omega 3 capsules. It took many years to get to where I am today as being natural did not happen overnight. My body feels good in the morning and throughout the day with no nose bleeds and steroid rages. When I made the transition to train in MMA, I did use testosterone and Anavar but more for the performance aspect. After MMA had finished, I competed in a natural bodybuilding federation and ended doing another 12-14 bodybuilding and fitness shows. I walked away from the pro qualifier show as I knew going back on steroids full time was the only way to achieve professional status. When I am 39, my plan is to use testosterone again but only for TRT (testosterone hormone therapy) since my hormone levels will never be the same again. I hope you enjoyed my story about my journey on what it took to gain over 55 lbs of muscle and to compete in over 20 bodybuilding shows. Coming off steroids and staying off is a constant battle for anyone. If you enjoyed this book, feel free to check out my other books on Amazon. Train smart, eat clean, and keep healthy!

ABOUT THE AUTHOR

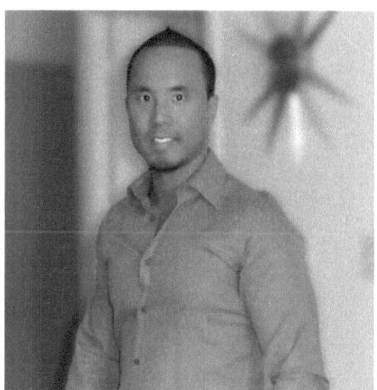

Paul Nam has been in the fitness industry and a personal trainer for over 23 years. He was chosen as one of Canada's Top Fitness Trainers for 2021 and 2022. He started bodybuilding at the age of 18 and became the Junior Mackenzie Bodybuilding Champion at 19. He has since competed in over 25 bodybuilding, fitness, and martial arts competitions. He has trained in Olympic style boxing, Brazilian jiu-jitsu, muay thai, and wrestling, and holds a black belt in taekwondo.

He owns a fitness studio in Toronto, builds mobile apps, writes books, and is bringing a few new fitness products to the world.

www.ingramcontent.com/pod-product-compliance
Lightning Source LLC
Chambersburg PA
CBHW050503290526
45786CB00006B/2416